Certification Logbook for Competencies in
Clinical Physiology Procedures

for Phase I MBBS Students

(As per Medical Council of India: Competency Based Undergraduate Curriculum for the Indian Medical Graduate)

Student's Name: _____

Roll No.: _____   Year/Session: _____

University Roll No.: _____

Name of the Institution: _____

This is to certify that the above student has been thoroughly trained in all the 13 clinical physiology procedures contained in this logbook and is henceforth competent to perform these procedures independently.

His/her overall performance is average/satisfactory/good/excellent.

_____

Signature of MBBS incharge

Submitted for University Examination in the year _____

_____

Signature of Professor and Head

Department of Physiology

Certification Logbook for Competencies in Clinical Physiology Procedures

for Phase I MBBS Students

(As per Medical Council of India: Competency Based Undergraduate Curriculum for the Indian Medical Graduate)

Compiled by

Jyoti Sethi MBBS MD
Professor and Head
Department of Physiology
Kalpana Chawla Government Medical College
Karnal, Haryana, India

Sharat Gupta MBBS MD
Associate Professor
Department of Physiology
Kalpana Chawla Government Medical College
Karnal, Haryana, India

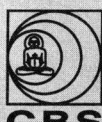

CBS

CBS Publishers & Distributors Pvt Ltd

New Delhi • Bengaluru • Chennai • Kochi • Kolkata • Mumbai
Bhopal • Bhubaneswar • Hyderabad • Jharkhand • Nagpur • Patna • Pune
• Uttarakhand • Dhaka (Bangladesh) • Kathmandu (Nepal)

Disclaimer:

We wish to clarify that this logbook should not be misunderstood as a clinical practical manual. It is to be meant to be used solely for certification purpose of the Phase I MBBS students in all the 13 clinical physiology procedures as per the CBME curriculum for the Indian Medical Graduate (IMG).

—Authors

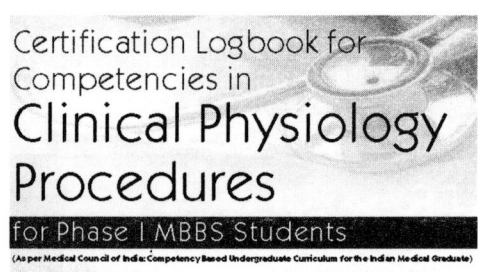

Certification Logbook for
Competencies in
**Clinical Physiology
Procedures**
for Phase I MBBS Students
(As per Medical Council of India: Competency Based Undergraduate Curriculum for the Indian Medical Graduate)

ISBN: 978-93-89565-76-8

Copyright © Authors and Publisher

First Edition: 2020

Published by Satish Kumar Jain and produced by Varun Jain for

CBS Publishers & Distributors Pvt Ltd
4819/XI Prahlad Street, 24 Ansari Road, Daryaganj, New Delhi 110 002, India.
Ph: 23289259, 23266861, 23266867 Website: www.cbspd.com
Fax: 011-23243014   e-mail: delhi@cbspd.com; cbspubs@airtelmail.in.
Corporate Office: 204 FIE, Industrial Area, Patparganj, Delhi 110 092

Ph: 4934 4934   Fax: 4934 4935   e-mail: publishing@cbspd.com; publicity@cbspd.com

Branches

• **Bengaluru:** Seema House 2975, 17th Cross, K.R. Road,
  Banasankari 2nd Stage, Bengaluru 560 070, Karnataka
  Ph: +91-80-26771678/79   Fax: +91-80-26771680   e-mail: bangalore@cbspd.com
• **Chennai:** 7, Subbaraya Street, Shenoy Nagar, Chennai 600 030, Tamil Nadu
  Ph: +91-44-26680620, 26681266   Fax: +91-44-42032115   e-mail: chennai@cbspd.com
• **Kochi:** 68/1534, 35, 36, Power House Road, Opp. KSEB, Kochi 682018, Kerala
  Ph: +91-484-4059061-65   Fax: +91-484-4059065   e-mail: kochi@cbspd.com
• **Kolkata:** 6/B, Ground Floor, Rameswar Shaw Road, Kolkata 700 014, West Bengal
  Ph: +91-33-22891126, 22891127, 22891128   e-mail: kolkata@cbspd.com
• **Mumbai:** 83-C, Dr E Moses Road, Worli, Mumbai 400018, Maharashtra
  Ph: +91-22-24902340/41   Fax: +91-22-24902342   e-mail: mumbai@cbspd.com

Representatives

• **Bhopal**	0-8319310552	• **Bhubaneswar**	0-9911037372	• **Hyderabad**	0-9885175004	• **Jharkhand**	0-9811541605
• **Nagpur**	0-9421945513	• **Patna**	0-9334159340	• **Pune**	0-9623451994	• **Uttarakhand**	0-9716462459
• **Dhaka (Bangladesh)**	01912-003485	• **Kathmandu (Nepal)**	977-9818742655				

Printed at Mudrak, Noida, UP, India

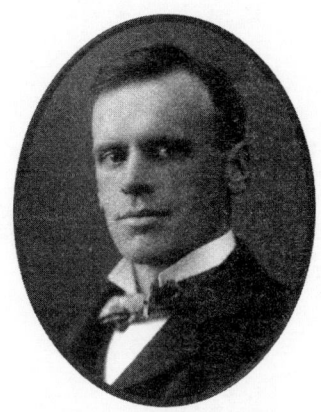

"Physiology of today is the medicine of tomorrow"
Dr Earnest Henry Starling
British Physiologist
(1866–1927)

Foreword

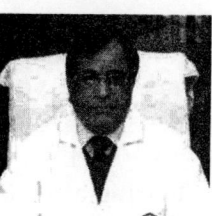

It gives me immense pleasure in writing the Foreword to this *manual Certification Logbook for Competencies in Clinical Physiology Procedures* authored by Prof Jyoti Sethi and Dr Sharat Gupta of Department of Physiology, Kalpana Chawla Government Medical College, Karnal. In 2014, I co-authored an article in *Medical Teachers* on **Medical Education in India: Current Challenges and the Way Forward.** We had emphasized the role of skill development during teaching and training of the medical students of India. I am happy to note that new curriculum brought out by the Board of Governors of Medical Council of India has given ample emphasis for Competency Based Medical Education (CBME). The new curriculum has been restructured and introduced from the academic year of 2019–20.

Physiology teaching during the undergraduate trainings as per CBME required 13 procedures to be perfected by each MBBS student needing certification by the Head, Department of Physiology, at the end of the session. To fulfil this requirement this manual will ensure quantification and assessment of students in clinical physiology in an objective and standardized manner leaving no chance of subjective bias. Further, the checklist for each procedure based on objective structured clinical examination (OSCE) has been provided. The assessment card provided in the logbook will facilitate the teacher to evaluate every student in a holistic manner with reference to his/her clinical skills and soft skills as a part of assessment of cognitive as well as communicative (AETCOM) domains.

What is most impressive about this *manual* is that it is comprehensive and as per the CBME requirements. I am sure that both medical teachers as well as students will benefit from the extensive efforts made by Prof Jyoti Sethi and Dr Sharat Gupta in bringing out this book in the shortest possible time.

Dr Surender Kashyap
Director
Kalpana Chawla Government Medical College
Karnal, Haryana

Foreword

It gives me immense pleasure to write the Foreword to this very useful and helpful *manual* conceptualized and brought out with the objective of standardizing the certification of certain competencies in clinical physiology, by two very dedicated and active teachers who are not only experts in their subject but are also motivated to implement the new CBME curriculum in letter and spirit.

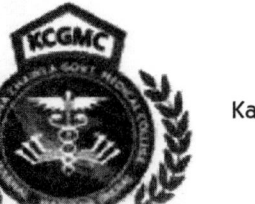

During attending the various faculty development programs, first as a learner in regional/ nodal centers and later as a resource faculty in different medical colleges, I observed that there was a lot of apprehension and speculation about the process of certification of competencies during the implementation of CBME curriculum. Nobody actually knew how to go about it and wanted some guidance about it. The common point of concern was as to how uniformity will be attained in various medical colleges across the country. This issue also came up in our discussion when we were preparing the First Prof time table at our institute. We strongly felt a need that there must be a standardization of the certification methods, otherwise it will compromise the essence of CBME. That was the moment when the idea of this *manual* was conceived by the authors and in record time they came out with the manual. Not only the effort but also the purpose is commendable. The USP of this manual is that the certification method has been framed by using reputed international clinical medicine textbooks as a reference.

I am sure this manual will prove to be very helpful for both teachers and students as it will help in reducing the subjective variation in certification and assessment of competencies. I also feel it will provide framework and motivation for designing such a manual for other specialties of the course.

Dr Himanshu Madaan
Professor, Department of Biochemistry
Dean Academics
Kalpana Chawla Government Medical College
Karnal, Haryana
and
Resource Faculty, MCI Regional Centre for
Faculty Development Programs, MAMC
New Delhi

Preface

The Board of Governors, Medical Council of India, has recently overhauled the age-old medical curriculum and has recently introduced the Competency Based Undergraduate Curriculum for the Indian medical graduate. This new curriculum has been designed keeping in mind the long pending demand of the experts of removing redundancy from the age-old curriculum and incorporating contemporary methodologies centred on acquisition of clinical skills by the MBBS students right from 1st year itself. It has also been felt that the student should be competent enough in certain basic clinical procedures being taught in the subject of human physiology, so that when they enter clinical ward/OPDs in 2nd year during clinical postings, they should be confident enough in performing basic clinical examination procedures on actual patients. A total of 13 such procedures in clinical physiology have been identified which need to be certified by the Professor and Head, department of physiology of medical colleges throughout India, for each student.

In this regard, the present logbook serves a dual purpose. On the one hand, it provides a ready reference which will guide the teachers as to how to assess the student in a holistic manner and on the other, at the same time it will also serve as a record book in which the data pertaining to the student certification and assessment can be entered.

We would also like to appraise our worthy colleagues and students that the contents of this book are open to constructive comments/review/suggestions. We will try to incorporate these in the future editions of this book. It is recommended that both the teachers as well as the students should read the corresponding guidelines given at the beginning of this book so that they can derive maximum benefit from this book.

Jyoti Sethi
Sharat Gupta

Acknowledgements

We bow our heads in gratitude before the Supreme Almighty for bestowing us with the intellect, resources, zeal and good luck; all of which are equally important for the success of any venture.

We are deeply indebted to our teachers who shaped the course of our academic careers with their assiduous pedagogy and meticulous guidance.

We are also grateful to our family members for being our pillar of strength and providing us their much needed love and moral support 24×7 during the preparation of this manuscript. Without them, this project would have never seen light of the day.

We extend our thanks to Dr Surender Kashyap, worthy Director, Kalpana Chawla Government Medical College, Karnal, Haryana, for providing a conducive academic environment and motivating us to fulfil his mission of making KCGMC a world class institution.

Our heartfelt gratitude is also due to Dr Himanshu Madaan, Professor of Biochemistry and Dean Academics, Kalpana Chawla Government Medical College, Karnal, Haryana, and Resource Faculty for MCI Regional Centre for Faculty Development Programme, Maulana Azad Medical College, New Delhi. It is her undulating passion in the field of medical education that has constantly motivated us to give our 100% efforts for the success of CBME curriculum.

Most importantly, our heartfelt thanks is also due to the entire team of CBS Publishers, especially Mr Satish Kumar Jain (CMD), Mr Varun Jain (Director), Mr YN Arjuna (Senior Vice President—Publishing, Editorial and Publicity), Mr Sumit Behl (Assistant Marketing Manager) and Ms Ritu Chawla (General Manager) for realising our potential and helping us in fruition of this manuscript.

Last but not the least, we are also thankful to all our students, past and present, because it is their presence that constantly inspires us to do better!

Jyoti Sethi
Sharat Gupta

Contents

Foreword by Dr Surender Kashyap vii

Foreword by Dr Himanshu Madaan viii

Preface ix

How to Use this Certification Logbook: A Guide for Teachers xvii

How to Perform Well in Competency Assessment: Some Tips for Students ... xviii

Cardiovascular System 1

Respiratory System 7

Neurophysiology 9

Index

Sr. No.	Competency No. and title of clinical procedure	Date	Page no.	Competent (Y/N)	Teacher's signature
CARDIOVASCULAR SYSTEM *No. of procedures that require certification: 03*					
1.	PY 5.12 Record pulse and blood pressure at rest in a volunteer.				
2.	PY 5.12 Record pulse and blood pressure in a volunteer in different grades of exercise.				
3.	PY 5.12 Record pulse and blood pressure in a volunteer during change of posture.				
RESPIRATORY SYSTEM *No. of procedures that require certification: 01*					
4.	PY 6.9 Demonstrate the correct clinical examination of respiratory system in a normal volunteer or simulated environment.				
NEUROPHYSIOLOGY *No. of procedures that require certification: 09*					
5.	PY 10.11 Demonstrate the correct clinical examination of higher functions of nervous system in a normal volunteer or simulated environment.				
6.	PY 10.11 Demonstrate the correct clinical examination of sensory system in a normal volunteer or simulated environment.				
7.	PY 10.11 Demonstrate the correct clinical examination of motor system in a normal volunteer or simulated environment.				
8.	PY 10.11 Demonstrate the correct clinical examination of reflexes in a normal volunteer or simulated environment.				
9.	PY 10.11 Demonstrate the correct clinical examination of cranial nerves in a normal volunteer or simulated environment.				
10.	PY 10.20 Demonstrate clinical testing of visual acuity, colour and field of vision in a normal volunteer or simulated environment				
11.	PY 10.20 Demonstrate hearing tests in a normal volunteer or simulated environment.				
12.	PY 10.20 Demonstrate testing of smell in a normal volunteer or simulated environment.				
13.	PY 10.20 Demonstrate taste sensation in a normal volunteer or simulated environment.				

How to Use this Certification Logbook
A Guide for Teachers

- The student should be given a detailed demonstration of the concerned practical skill in the laboratory on a normal subject via DOAP (demonstrate observe assist perform) method, during the routine practical classes.
- The student must then practice that procedure under close monitoring by the teacher concerned until the teacher is sure that the student is competent to perform these procedures independently.
- Thereafter, an assessment of the practical skills may be carried out based on the corresponding checklist provided with each procedure. This checklist has been prepared in accordance with the objective structured clinical examination (OSCE) pattern.
- The teachers are required to give a score from 1 to 5 to the student for each of the five parameters, i.e. behaviour towards the patient, communication skills, confidence level, procedural skills (i.e. systematic approach during the procedure) and knowledge level. A suggestive scale has been given to help the teachers in deciding the score to be awarded for each skill.
- The scoring system has been designed to assess the cognitive domain as well as the behavioural domain of the students (or AETCOM, i.e. Attitude, Ethics and Communication module) as per CBME curriculum.
- The cumulative total of the score of all the above five parameters will then be compared against a final assessment scale to grade the overall performance of the student in each procedure as **unsatisfactory** (final score <10), **satisfactory** (score 11–19) and **excellent** (final score 20 and above).
- A student needs to obtain a minimum final score of 10 (i.e. satisfactory) in each procedure in order to be declared competent for that procedure.
- The student whose final score is <10 (i.e. unsatisfactory) in any competency should be reassessed by the teacher until the score improves.
- Based on the steps missed/performed by the student as per the checklist, the teachers can share their feedback on the student's performance during the assessment, focussing on his/her individual strengths as well as weaknesses in each procedure, in the "remarks" section.
- Upon successful completion of all the 13 procedures, the Professor and Head of the concerned physiology department of that institution will give a final certification to each student.
- **Note:** For the ease of our colleagues, we have also provided sample proformas for each of the 13 procedures in which the students can record their findings. The format of these proformas has been prepared according to standardised techniques outlined in reputed international clinical medicine textbooks. However, it may be noted that these proformas are merely suggestive; the teachers should feel free to customise them as per their institute's norms.
- **Suggested reading for clinical procedures:**
  1. *Bates' Guide to Physical Examination and History Taking*, 12th edition, Lynn S Bickley, Wolters Kluwer Publishers.
  2. *Hutchinson's Clinical Methods: An Integrated Approach to Clinical Practice*, 24th edition, Elsevier Publishers.
  3. *Macleod's Clinical Examination*, 13th edition. Churchill Livingstone Publishers.

How to Perform Well in Competency Assessment
Some Tips for Students

- **General tips:**
  1. Dress appropriately; formal wear is the best.
  2. ALWAYS wear your apron.
  3. Listen carefully to your examiner and try to answer with politeness, confidence and common sense. DO NOT argue at any point.
  4. Be confident; BUT don't be overconfident or underconfident.

- **Approach towards the subject/patient:**
  1. ALWAYS GREET the subject before you start examining.
  2. Be sure to obtain subject's consent (written/verbal) prior to examination.
  3. It is advisable to converse with subject in his/her local language and know his name, age, background, job, etc. before you start the procedure. This will help you in developing a good rapport with the subject and ensure his/her cooperation during the procedure.
  4. Be very clear while giving instructions to your subject and also explain him/her the procedure in brief. Try not to seem confused.
  5. Before performing any procedure, be sure to crosscheck that he/she has fully understood the same. DON'T START the procedure until you are ABSOLUTELY SURE that he/she has understood your instructions.
  6. Stop the procedure at any point if you feel that the subject is feeling uneasy and uncomfortable. Reassure him/her and restart.
  7. Always thank your subject at the end of the procedure.

- **Methodology:**
  1. Before starting the examination, ensure that you have all the necessary equipment and it is in working condition.
  2. Always remember "The eye sees what the mind knows"; thus it is important that you should always plan the steps beforehand and then perform the required steps in a proper sequence so that you don't miss any of the steps.
  3. You should have "a damsel's hand (firm yet gentle) and an aquiline (eagle like) vision" during the procedure.

- **Data compilation and presentation of results:**
  1. Record the observations and express the results in proper units.
  2. Document your findings in a neat and tidy manner. It is better to avoid cutting and overwriting as much as possible.
  3. For final result/interpretation purpose, the student should compare the findings/values obtained in the subject with the standard parameters.
  4. The final result should always be reported in a proper format.
     - *For example, the result for BP may be given as follows:*
       The BP of the given subject is… mmHg and it is within normal limits/abnormally high/abnormally low.

CARDIOVASCULAR SYSTEM

PROCEDURE 1

AIM: PY 5.12: Record pulse and blood pressure at rest in a volunteer.

Number of times this skill needs to be done to be certified for independent performance = 01.

Sr. No.	Steps to be performed sequentially	Performed (Y/N)
Checklist for examination of radial pulse		
i.	Stands on the right side of the patient and explains the procedure in subject's own language.	
ii.	Supports the subject's right arm and holds it in proper position (semi-prone and semi-flexed).	
iii.	Places 3 fingers (index, middle and ring finger) on the radial artery.	
iv.	Counts the pulse rate for 1 full minute.	
v.	Determines all other important characteristics of pulse.	
vi.	Expresses the result in proper format.	
Checklist for arterial blood pressure (BP)		
i.	Keeps the BP apparatus at the level of the heart and explains the procedure in subject's own language.	
ii.	Checks the BP apparatus for any zero error and/or leakage in mercury bulb or cuff.	
iii.	Exposes the arm up to the shoulder or ensures bare minimum clothing on arm.	
iv.	Wraps the BP cuff firmly around the upper arm, keeping its lower edge 2.5 cms above antecubital crease. Checks that it is snugly fit.	
v.	Performs palpatory method first and notes the reading.	
vi.	Re-inflates the cuff and raises the mercury column around 30 mmHg more than the reading obtained by palpatory method.	
vii.	Performs auscultatory method.	
viii.	Takes 3 separate readings of SBP and DBP at 2 minutes intervals and takes their average to obtain final reading.	
ix.	Expresses the result in proper format.	

ASSESSMENT CARD FOR PROCEDURE 1

Sr. No.	Attributes to be assessed	Score (1–5)*
i.	Behavioural skill	
ii.	Communication skill	
iii.	Confidence level	
iv.	Procedural skill	
v.	Knowledge level	
	Grand total (out of 25)	

*Note: The teacher may decide the score as given below:

Below average	Average	Good	Very good	Excellent
1	2	3	4	5

Overall rating of the candidate will be done based on the grand total obtained above and will be finally assessed as follows:

Grand total	Overall rating
9 or less	Unsatisfactory
10–19	Satisfactory
20 and above	Excellent

Teacher's remarks:

_____

_____

_____

_____

_____

Signature of teacher

PROCEDURE 2

AIM: PY 5.12 Record pulse and blood pressure in a volunteer in different grades of exercise.

Number of times this skill needs to be done to be certified for independent performance = 01.

Sr. No.	Steps to be performed sequentially	Performed (Y/N)
	Checklist for procedure	
i.	Stands on the right side of the patient and explains the procedure in subject's own language.	
ii.	Checks the BP apparatus for any zero error and/or leakage in mercury bulb or cuff.	
iii.	Asks the subject to observe complete mental and physical rest for at least 5 minutes.	
iv.	Records the pulse and BP of the subject at rest.	
v.	Without removing the BP cuff, asks the subject to perform exercise of pre-determined intensity (i.e. mild/moderate or severe).	
vi.	Records the pulse and BP immediately after exercise and at regular predetermined time intervals.	
vii.	Compares the pre- and post-exercise pulse and BP values and expresses the result in proper format.	

ASSESSMENT CARD FOR PROCEDURE 2

Sr. No.	Attributes to be assessed	Score (1–5)*
i.	Behavioural skill	
ii.	Communication skill	
iii.	Confidence level	
iv.	Procedural skill	
v.	Knowledge level	
	Grand total (out of 25)	

*Note: The teacher may decide the score as given below:

Below average	Average	Good	Very good	Excellent
1	2	3	4	5

Overall rating of the candidate will be done based on the grand total obtained above and will be finally assessed as follows:

Grand total	Overall rating
9 or less	Unsatisfactory
10–19	Satisfactory
20 and above	Excellent

Teacher's remarks:

_____

_____

_____

_____

_____

Signature of teacher

PROCEDURE 3

AIM: PY 5.12 Record pulse and blood pressure in a volunteer during change of posture.

Number of times this skill needs to be done to be certified for independent performance = 01.

Checklist for procedure		
Sr. No.	*Steps to be performed sequentially*	*Performed (Y/N)*
i.	Stands on the right side of the patient and explains the procedure in subject's own language.	
ii.	Checks the BP apparatus for any zero error and/or leakage in mercury bulb or cuff.	
iii.	Asks the patient to lie down supine on a couch and records the pulse and BP by both palpatory and auscultatory method.	
iv.	Without removing the BP cuff, immediately asks the subject to stand up quickly without support.	
v.	Records the pulse and BP immediately upon standing and after 3 minutes of standing.	
vi.	Compares the pulse and BP values obtained in supine and standing posture and expresses the results in proper format.	

ASSESSMENT CARD FOR PROCEDURE 3

Sr. No.	Attributes to be assessed	Score (1–5)*
i.	Behavioural skill	
ii.	Communication skill	
iii.	Confidence level	
iv.	Procedural skill	
v.	Knowledge level	
	Grand total (out of 25)	

*Note: The teacher may decide the score as given below:

Below average	Average	Good	Very good	Excellent
1	2	3	4	5

Overall rating of the candidate will be done based on the grand total obtained above and will be finally assessed as follows:

Grand total	Overall rating
9 or less	Unsatisfactory
10–19	Satisfactory
20 and above	Excellent

Teacher's remarks:

_____

_____

_____

_____

_____

Signature of teacher

RESPIRATORY SYSTEM

PROCEDURE 4

AIM: PY 6.9 Demonstrate the correct clinical examination of respiratory system in a normal volunteer or simulated environment.

Number of times this skill needs to be done to be certified for independent performance = 01.

Sr. No.	Steps to be performed sequentially	Performed (Y/N)
	Checklist for procedure	
i.	Stands on the right side of the patient and explains the procedure briefly in subject's own language.	
ii.	Takes a brief and relevant history of the patient before starting the physical examination.	
iii.	Performs the general physical examination of the patient.	
iv.	Starts respiratory system examination by inspection of thorax.	
v.	Performs palpation of thorax.	
vi.	Performs percussion of thorax.	
vii.	Performs auscultation of thorax.	
viii.	Records the findings in a proper format.	

ASSESSMENT CARD FOR PROCEDURE 4

Sr. No.	Attributes to be assessed	Score (1–5)*
i.	Behavioural skill	
ii.	Communication skill	
iii.	Confidence level	
iv.	Procedural skill	
v.	Knowledge level	
	Grand total (out of 25)	

Note: The teacher may decide the score as given below:

Below average	Average	Good	Very good	Excellent
1	2	3	4	5

Overall rating of the candidate will be done based on the grand total obtained above and will be finally assessed as follows:

Grand total	Overall rating
9 or less	Unsatisfactory
10–19	Satisfactory
20 and above	Excellent

Teacher's remarks:

_____

_____

_____

_____

_____

Signature of teacher

NEUROPHYSIOLOGY

PROCEDURE 5

AIM: PY 10.11 Demonstrate the correct clinical examination of higher functions of nervous system in a normal volunteer or simulated environment.

Number of times this skill needs to be done to be certified for independent performance = 01.

Checklist for procedure		
Sr. No.	Steps to be performed sequentially	Performed (Y/N)
i.	Explains the procedure in brief in subject's own language.	
ii.	Takes a brief and relevant history of the subject.	
iii.	Checks and notes down the level of consciousness, orientation and cooperation level of subject.	
iv.	Checks and notes down the overall appearance (hygiene), behaviour and emotional state of subject.	
v.	Notes whether the subject has any illusion, delusion and/or hallucination or not.	
vi.	Tests the memory (recent and past) of the subject.	
vii.	Tests the subject's intelligence levels, speech and handedness.	
viii.	Records the findings in a proper format.	

ASSESSMENT CARD FOR PROCEDURE 5

Sr. No.	Attributes to be assessed	Score (1–5)*
i.	Behavioural skill	
ii.	Communication skill	
iii.	Confidence level	
iv.	Procedural skill	
v.	Knowledge level	
	Grand total (out of 25)	

*Note: The teacher may decide the score as given below:

Below average	Average	Good	Very good	Excellent
1	2	3	4	5

Overall rating of the candidate will be done based on the grand total obtained above and will be finally assessed as follows:

Grand total	Overall rating
9 or less	Unsatisfactory
10–19	Satisfactory
20 and above	Excellent

Teacher's remarks:

_____

_____

_____

_____

_____

Signature of teacher

PROCEDURE 6

AIM: PY 10.11 Demonstrate the correct clinical examination of sensory system in a normal volunteer or simulated environment.

Number of times this skill needs to be done to be certified for independent performance = 01.

Sr.No.	Steps to be performed sequentially	Performed (Y/N)
	Checklist for procedure	
i.	Stands on the right side of the patient and explains the procedure very clearly in subject's own language.	
ii.	Asks the subject to keep his/her eyes closed throughout the test and turn his/her face towards the opposite side.	
iii.	Performs tests for dorsal column sensations.	
iv.	Performs tests for spinothalamic tract sensations.	
v.	Performs tests for stereognosis and graphesthesia.	
vi.	Compares the findings on both sides and records the findings in a proper format.	

ASSESSMENT CARD FOR PROCEDURE 6

Sr. No.	Attributes to be assessed	Score (1–5)*
i.	Behavioural skill	
ii.	Communication skill	
iii.	Confidence level	
iv.	Procedural skill	
v.	Knowledge level	
	Grand total (out of 25)	

*Note: The teacher may decide the score as given below:

Below average	Average	Good	Very good	Excellent
1	2	3	4	5

Overall rating of the candidate will be done based on the grand total obtained above and will be finally assessed as follows:

Grand total	Overall rating
9 or less	Unsatisfactory
10–19	Satisfactory
20 and above	Excellent

Teacher's remarks:

_____

_____

_____

_____

_____

Signature of teacher

PROCEDURE 7

AIM: PY 10.11 Demonstrate the correct clinical examination of motor system in a normal volunteer or simulated environment.

Number of times this skill needs to be done to be certified for independent performance = 01.

Sr. No.	Steps to be performed sequentially	Performed (Y/N)
	Checklist for procedure	
i.	Stands on the right side of the patient and explains the procedure very clearly in subject's own language.	
ii.	Asks the subject to expose the upper/lower limbs.	
iii.	Notes the bulk of muscles.	
iv.	Estimates the muscle tone.	
v.	Tests and grades the strength (power) of muscles.	
vi.	Notes the gait of subject.	
vii.	Compares the observations of upper and lower limbs on both sides and records the findings in proper format.	

ASSESSMENT CARD FOR PROCEDURE 7

Sr. No.	Attributes to be assessed	Score (1–5)*
i.	Behavioural skill	
ii.	Communication skill	
iii.	Confidence level	
iv.	Procedural skill	
v.	Knowledge level	
	Grand total (out of 25)	

Note: The teacher may decide the score as given below:

Below average	Average	Good	Very good	Excellent
1	2	3	4	5

Overall rating of the candidate will be done based on the grand total obtained above and will be finally assessed as follows:

Grand total	Overall rating
9 or less	Unsatisfactory
10–19	Satisfactory
20 and above	Excellent

Teacher's remarks:

_____

_____

_____

_____

_____

Signature of teacher

PROCEDURE 8

AIM: PY 10.11 Demonstrate the correct clinical examination of reflexes in a normal volunteer or simulated environment.

Number of times this skill needs to be done to be certified for independent performance = 01.

	Checklist for procedure	
Sr. No.	Steps to be performed sequentially	Performed (Y/N)
i.	Stands on the right side of the patient and explains the procedure very clearly in subject's own language.	
ii.	Asks the subject to expose the upper/lower limbs and also ensures that the subject is fully relaxed with head turned in opposite direction.	
iii.	Correctly elicits biceps reflex.	
iv.	Correctly elicits triceps reflex.	
v.	Correctly elicits supinator reflex.	
vi.	Correctly elicits knee jerk.	
vii.	Correctly elicits ankle jerk.	
viii.	Correctly elicits jaw jerk.	
ix.	Correctly elicits plantar reflex.	
x.	Asks the patient to perform Jandressik's manoeuvre in case of non-elicitation of deep tendon reflexes.	
xi.	Compares the results on both sides and records the findings in proper format.	

ASSESSMENT CARD FOR PROCEDURE 8

Sr. No.	Attributes to be assessed	Score (1–5)*
i.	Behavioural skill	
ii.	Communication skill	
iii.	Confidence level	
iv.	Procedural skill	
v.	Knowledge level	
	Grand total (out of 25)	

Note: The teacher may decide the score as given below:

Below average	Average	Good	Very good	Excellent
1	2	3	4	5

Overall rating of the candidate will be done based on the grand total obtained above and will be finally assessed as follows:

Grand total	Overall rating
9 or less	Unsatisfactory
10–19	Satisfactory
20 and above	Excellent

Teacher's remarks:

_____

_____

_____

_____

_____

Signature of teacher

PROCEDURE 9

AIM: PY 10.11 Demonstrate the correct clinical examination of cranial nerves in a normal volunteer or simulated environment.

Number of times this skill needs to be done to be certified for independent performance = 01.

Sr. No.	Steps to be performed sequentially	Performed (Y/N)
	Checklist for procedure	
i.	Stands on the right side of the patient and explains the procedure very clearly in subject's own language.	
	Checklist for Cranial Nerve I	
i	Performs tests for olfaction.	
	Checklist for Cranial Nerve II	
i.	Performs tests for distant vision.	
ii.	Performs tests for near vision.	
iii.	Performs tests for colour vision.	
iv.	Checks field of vision.	
	Checklist for Cranial Nerves III, IV and VI	
i.	Checks the functioning of extraocular muscles.	
ii.	Elicits direct and indirect light reflex.	
iii.	Elicits accommodation reflex.	
	Checklist for Cranial Nerve V	
i.	Elicits corneal and conjunctival reflexes.	
ii.	Eliciting mandibular reflex and checks muscles of mastication.	
	Checklist for Cranial Nerve VII	
i.	Elicits the motor functions of facial nerve.	
ii.	Elicits the sensory (taste) function of facial nerve.	
	Checklist for Cranial Nerve VIII	
i.	Elicits whisper test.	
ii.	Elicits tuning fork tests.	
	Checklist for Cranial Nerves IX, X, XI and XII	
i.	Elicits palatal and pharyngeal reflexes.	
ii.	Checks the spinal part of accessory nerve.	
iii.	Checks the movements of tongue.	
iv.	Compares the results obtained for all cranial nerves and reports the observations in proper format.	

ASSESSMENT CARD FOR PROCEDURE 9

Sr. No.	Attributes to be assessed	Score (1–5)*
i.	Behavioural skill	
ii.	Communication skill	
iii.	Confidence level	
iv.	Procedural skill	
v.	Knowledge level	
	Grand total (out of 25)	

*Note: The teacher may decide the score as given below:

Below average	Average	Good	Very good	Excellent
1	2	3	4	5

Overall rating of the candidate will be done based on the grand total obtained above and will be finally assessed as follows:

Grand total	Overall rating
9 or less	Unsatisfactory
10–19	Satisfactory
20 and above	Excellent

Teacher's remarks:

_____

_____

_____

_____

_____

Signature of teacher

PROCEDURE 10

AIM: PY 10.20 Demonstrate clinical testing of visual acuity, colour and field of vision in a normal volunteer or simulated environment.

Number of times this skill needs to be done to be certified for independent performance = 01.

Sr. No.	Steps to be performed sequentially	Performed (Y/N)
i.	Explains the procedure to the subject in his/her own language.	
ii.	Asks the subject to close opposite eye during the test.	
iii.	Correctly tests the distant vision of the subject.	
iv.	Correctly tests the near vision of the subject.	
v.	Correctly tests the colour vision of the subject.	
vi.	Performs confrontation test first for visual field.	
vii.	Performs perimetry.	
viii.	Compares the result on both sides and reports the observations in proper format.	

Checklist for procedure

ASSESSMENT CARD FOR PROCEDURE 10

Sr. No.	Attributes to be assessed	Score (1–5)*
i.	Behavioural skill	
ii.	Communication skill	
iii.	Confidence level	
iv.	Procedural skill	
v.	Knowledge level	
	Grand total (out of 25)	

*Note: The teacher may decide the score as given below:

Below average	Average	Good	Very good	Excellent
1	2	3	4	5

Overall rating of the candidate will be done based on the grand total obtained above and will be finally assessed as follows:

Grand total	Overall rating
9 or less	Unsatisfactory
10–19	Satisfactory
20 and above	Excellent

Teacher's remarks:

_____

_____

_____

_____

_____

Signature of teacher

PROCEDURE 11

AIM: PY 10.20 Demonstrate hearing tests in a normal volunteer or simulated environment.

Number of times this skill needs to be done to be certified for independent performance = 01.

Sr. No.	Steps to be performed sequentially	Performed (Y/N)
	Checklist for procedure	
i.	Explains the procedure to the subject in his/her own language. And also ensures that there is no unnecessary background noise in the room.	
ii.	Asks the subject to close his opposite external auditory meatus with his/her finger.	
iii.	Elicits whisper test.	
iv.	Selects the tuning fork of correct frequency for tuning fork tests, i.e. 256 Hz.	
v.	Correctly performs Rinne's test.	
vi.	Correctly performs Weber's test.	
vii.	Correctly performs Schwabach's test.	
viii.	Compares the result on both sides and records the findings in proper format.	

ASSESSMENT CARD FOR PROCEDURE 11

Sr. No.	Attributes to be assessed	Score (1–5)*
i.	Behavioural skill.	
ii.	Communication skill.	
iii.	Confidence level.	
iv.	Procedural skill.	
v.	Knowledge level.	
	Grand total (out of 25)	

*Note: The teacher may decide the score as given below:

Below average	Average	Good	Very good	Excellent
1	2	3	4	5

Overall rating of the candidate will be done based on the grand total obtained above and will be finally assessed as follows:

Grand total	Overall rating
9 or less	Unsatisfactory
10–19	Satisfactory
20 and above	Excellent

Teacher's remarks:

_____

_____

_____

_____

_____

Signature of teacher

PROCEDURE 12

AIM: PY 10.20 Demonstrate testing of smell in a normal volunteer or simulated environment.

Number of times this skill needs to be done to be certified for independent performance = 01.

Sr. No.	Steps to be performed sequentially	Performed (Y/N)
	Checklist for procedure	
i.	Explains the procedure to the subject in his/her own language.	
ii.	Checks that the nostrils are patent by compressing one nostril and asking the subject to sniff through the other.	
iii.	Asks the subject to close his/her eyes and also occlude opposite nostril.	
iv.	Exposes the subject to familiar odours and asks him/her to identify these odours one by one.	
v.	Repeats the procedure for other nostril and reports the findings in proper format.	

ASSESSMENT CARD FOR PROCEDURE 12

Sr. No.	Attributes to be assessed	Score (1–5)*
i.	Behavioural skill	
ii.	Communication skill	
iii.	Confidence level	
iv.	Procedural skill	
v.	Knowledge level	
	Grand total (out of 25)	

*Note: The teacher may decide the score as given below:

Below average	Average	Good	Very good	Excellent
1	2	3	4	5

Overall rating of the candidate will be done based on the grand total obtained above and will be finally assessed as follows:

Grand total	Overall rating
9 or less	Unsatisfactory
10–19	Satisfactory
20 and above	Excellent

Teacher's remarks:

_____

_____

_____

_____

_____

Signature of teacher

PROCEDURE 13

AIM: PY 10.20 Demonstrate taste sensation in a normal volunteer or simulated environment.

Number of times this skill needs to be done to be certified for independent performance = 01.

Sr. No.	Steps to be performed sequentially	Performed (Y/N)
	Checklist for procedure	
i.	Explains the procedure to the subject in his/her own language.	
ii.	Asks the subject not to speak during the test and provides him four cards to indicate the type of taste being tested.	
iii.	Asks the subject to thoroughly rinse his/her mouth before the procedure and also after every new taste sample.	
iv.	Checks for perception of different taste modalities and reports the findings in a proper format.	

ASSESSMENT CARD FOR PROCEDURE 13

Sr. No.	Attributes to be assessed	Score (1–5)*
i.	Behavioural skill	
ii.	Communication skill	
iii.	Confidence level	
iv.	Procedural skill	
v.	Knowledge level	
	Grand total (out of 25)	

***Note:** The teacher may decide the score as given below:

Below average	Average	Good	Very good	Excellent
1	2	3	4	5

Overall Rating of the candidate will be done based on the grand total obtained above and will be finally assessed as follows:

Grand total	Overall rating
9 or less	Unsatisfactory
10–19	Satisfactory
20 and above	Excellent

Teacher's remarks:

_____

_____

_____

_____

_____

Signature of teacher

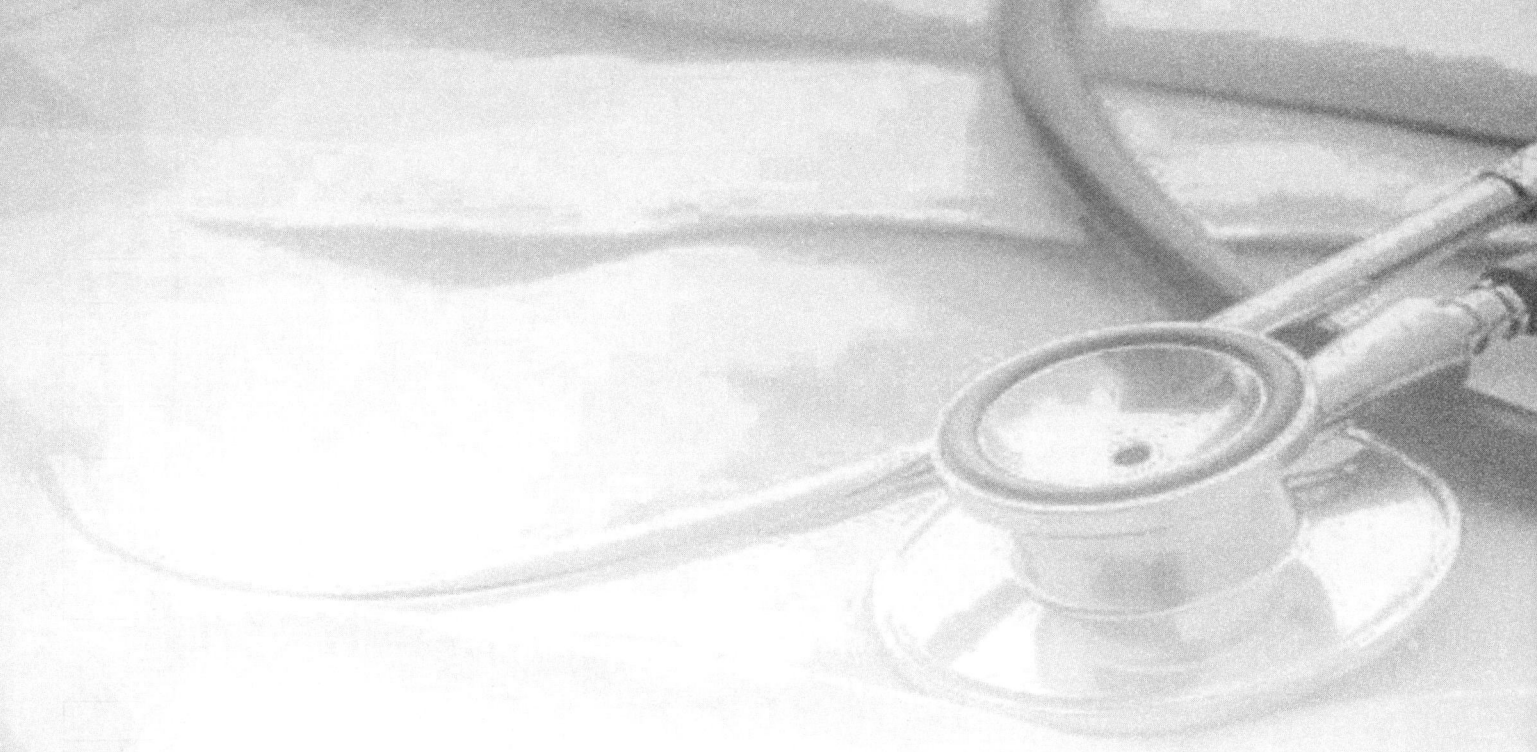

Sample Proformas to be Used by Students for Reporting Findings/Observations of Clinical Procedures for Certification

PROFORMA FOR PROCEDURE 1

Subject's name: Date:

Age:

Gender: Male/Female

Observations:

Examination of radial pulse:

    Rate: _____ per minute.

    Rhythm: Regularly regular/regularly irregular/irregularly irregular.

    Volume: Good/Low/High

    Any special character: No/Yes (if yes, please specify) _____

    Condition of vessel wall: Palpable/Not palpable

    Equality on both sides: Equal/Unequal

    Radiofemoral delay: Present/Absent/Not elicited

    Other peripheral pulses: Present/Absent

Recording of BP:

    Zero error in instrument (if any): _____
    Palpatory method: Systolic BP: _____ mmHg.
    Auscultatory method:

	Reading 1	Reading 2	Reading 3
Systolic BP (mmHg)			
Diastolic BP (mmHg)			

Result/Interpretation:

Signature of Student   *Signature of teacher*

Note:

Blood pressure classification for adults as per JNC 7 guidelines of American Society of Hypertension.

Category	Systolic BP (mmHg)	Diastolic BP (mmHg)
Normal	<120	<80
Prehypertension	120–139	80–89
Stage 1 hypertension	140–159	90–99
Stage 2 hypertension	≥160	≥100

Source: https://www.nhlbi.nih.gov/files/docs/guidelines/jnc7full.pdf

PROFORMA FOR PROCEDURE 2

Subject's name: Date:

Age:

Gender: Male/Female

Observations:

Intensity of exercise*: Mild/Moderate/Severe

	Pulse rate (beats per minute)	Blood pressure (mmHg)	
		Systolic	Diastolic
At rest (baseline values)			
Immediately after exercise			
5 minutes after exercise			
10 minutes after exercise			

Result/Interpretation:

Signature of student   *Signature of teacher*

*Intensity of exercise to be decided as per guidelines given by American Heart Association as follows:

1. Calculate the Maximum Heart Rate (MHR) of the subject using the following formula:

$$MHR = 220 - age \text{ (in years)}$$

2. Intensity of the exercise can then be gauged from the following table

Heart rate at the end of exercise	Exercise intensity
<50% of MHR	Mild
50–70% of MHR	Moderate
>70% of MHR	Severe

Source: Official website of American Heart Association:

https://www.heart.org/en/healthy-living/fitness/fitness-basics/target-heart-rates

PROFORMA FOR PROCEDURE 3

Subject's name: Date:

Age:

Gender: Male/Female

Observations:

	Pulse rate (beats per minute)	Blood Pressure (mmHg)	
		Systolic BP	Diastolic BP
Lying down posture			
Immediately upon standing			
3 minutes after standing			

Result/Interpretation:

Signature of student   *Signature of teacher*

PROFORMA FOR PROCEDURE 4

Subject's name: Date:

Age:

Gender: Male/Female

Occupation:

Does the subject smoke (yes/no):

If yes, then how many packets of cigarettes per day and since how many years:

Brief relevant history:

General physical examination:

General condition of patient:

Pallor:	Present/Absent
Icterus:	Present/Absent
Cyanosis:	Present/Absent
Clubbing:	Present/Absent
Edema feet:	Present/Absent
Cervical/axillary lymphadenopathy:	Present/Absent

Vitals:

Temperature:	_____°F
Pulse rate:	_____ per min.
BP:	_____ mmHg.
Respiratory rate:	_____ per min.

Respiratory System Examination

INSPECTION

Shape of chest: Normal/abnormal (specify)

Movement of chest: Symmetrical/asymmetrical

Type of breathing: Abdomino-throacic/thoraco-abdominal

Any visible veins/scar mark on chest: No/Yes

PALPATION

Local temperature: Normal/raised

Any area of tenderness: No/Yes (specify)

Position of trachea: Midline/_____ sided

Chest expansion: _____ cm

Vocal fremitus: Present/Absent

PERCUSSION

Chest resonance: Non-resonant/resonant/hyper-resonant

Vocal resonance: Present/Absent

Liver dullness: Starts from _____ right intercostal space/absent

Cardiac dullness: Starts from _____ left intercostal space/absent

AUSCULTATION

Breath sounds: Bronchial/Vesicular

Adventitious sounds: Absent/Present (specify type and location)

Vocal resonance: Present/Absent

Result/Interpretation:

Signature of student   *Signature of teacher*

PROFORMA FOR PROCEDURE 5

Subject's name: Date:

Age:

Gender: Male/Female

Occupation:

Brief relevant history:

Higher Functions Assessment

1. Level of consciousness of subject: Alert/Semi-conscious/Unconscious

2. General appearance: Normal/Abnormal

3. Behaviour: Co-operative/Uncooperative

4. Emotional state: Normal/Agitated/Depressed/other

5. Oriented with respect to time, place and person: Well-oriented/Disoriented

6. Any illusion/delusion/hallucination: Yes/No

   (*If yes, then please describe*)

7. Memory (recent and past events):   Normal/Abnormal

8. Intelligence: Normal/Subnormal

9. Speech: Normal/Abnormal

   (*If abnormal, describe the type of abnormality*)

10. Handedness: Left handed/Right handed

Result/Interpretations:

Signature of student   *Signature of teacher*

PROFORMA FOR PROCEDURE 6

Subject's name: Date:

Age:

Gender: Male/Female

Sensory System Assessment

Sensations	Left side	Right side
Dorsal column sensations (perceived/not perceived)		
Pressure		
Fine touch		
Proprioception		
Tactile localisation		
Two-point discrimination		
Vibration		
Anterolateral spinothalamic tract sensations		
Crude touch		
Pain (to be rated as per VAS)*		
Temperature		
Synthetic sensations		
Stereognosis		
Graphasthesia		

Result/Interpretation:

Signature of student   *Signature of teacher*

* The grading of pain perception should be done as per Visual Analog Scale (VAS). The subject is asked to point out a number to indicate the intensity of pain felt from the scale below:

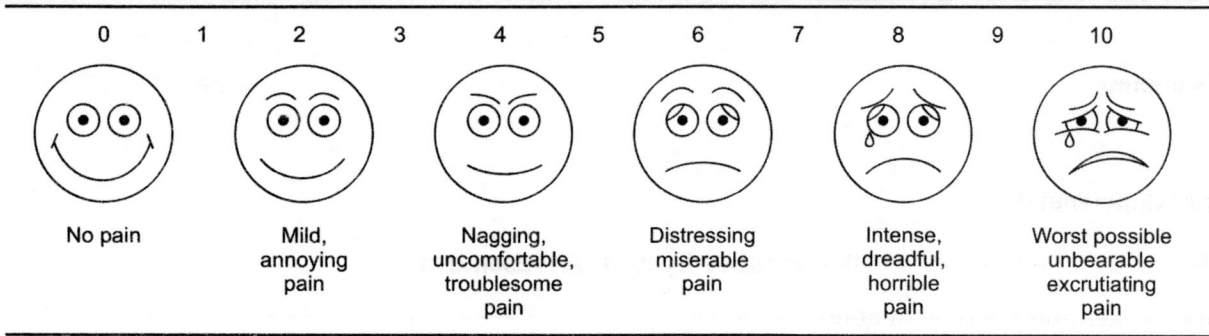

Source: https://operativeneurosurgery.com/doku.php?id=visual_analog_scale

PROFORMA FOR PROCEDURE 7

Subject's name: Date:

Age:

Gender: Male/Female

Gait of the subject: Normal/Abnormal

(If abnormal, mention the type of abnormality).

Motor System Examination

Characteristic	Left side	Right side
1. Bulk of muscle		
a. Mid-arm circumference	cm	cm
b. Mid-thigh circumference	cm	cm
c. Mid-calf circumference	cm	cm
2. Muscle tone (normal/hypotonia/hypertonia)		
a. Upper limbs		
b. Lower limbs		
3. Power of muscles (provide grades)*		
a. Hand		
b. Shoulder and arm		
c. Hip and thigh		
d. Leg		
4. Any involuntary movements (Y/N)		

Result/Interpretation

Signature of student   *Signature of teacher*

* Gradation of muscle power may be done as per Medical Research Council (MRC) scale for muscle strength as follows:

Grade	Description
Grade 0	Complete paralysis.
Grade 1	No movement are possible, only a flicker of contraction is present.
Grade 2	Muscle power can be detected only when effect of gravity is removed by making appropriate postural adjustments.
Grade 3	The limb can be held against gravity but not against passive resistance applied by examiner.
Grade 4	Movements are possible against examiner's resistance; but are weak.
Grade 5	Normal muscle power both against gravity and against examiner's resistance.

Source: http://medicalcriteria.com/web/neuromrc/

PROFORMA FOR PROCEDURE 8

Subject's name: Date:

Age:

Gender: Male/Female

Reflexes Examination

Reflex	Left side	Right side
Plantar reflex (normal/absent/abnormal)		
Deep reflexes (provide grades for each)*		
Biceps jerk		
Triceps jerk		
Supinator jerk		
Knee jerk		
Ankle jerk		
Jaw jerk		

Jendrassik's (Reinforcement) manoeuvre required: Y/N.

(If yes, please mention the jerk for which it was required)

Result/Interpretation:

Signature of student   *Signature of teacher*

* Reflexes should be graded as follows:

Grade	Written as	Description
0	0	Absent
1	+	Present but weak
2	++	Normal (brisk)
3	+++	Very brisk
4	++++	Clonus

Source: *Bates' Guide to Physical Examination and History Taking*, 12th edition, pp. 758, 773.

PROFORMA FOR PROCEDURE 9

Subject's name: Date:

Age:

Gender: Male/Female

Cranial Nerves (CN) Examination

(Result to be reported as normal/abnormal or present/absent as appropriate)

Tests performed	Left side	Right side
Olfactory nerve (CN I)		
i. Smell sensitivity		
Optic nerve (CN II)		
i. Visual acuity		
ii. Colour vision		
iii. Field of vision		
Occulomotor, Trochlear and Abducent Nerves (CN III, IV and VI)		
i. Pupil (size, shape)		
ii. Ptosis, squint		
iii. Ocular movements		
iv. Pupillary light reflexes		
v. Accommodation reflex		
Trigeminal nerve (CN V)		
i. Corneal and conjunctival reflexes		
ii. Mandibular reflex (muscles of mastication)		
Facial nerve (CN VII)		
i. Facial appearance		
ii. Taste sensation (ant 1/3rd of tongue)		
iii. Muscles of face		
iv. Schirmer's test (for lacrimation)		
Vestibulo-cochlear nerve (CN VIII): Cochlear division		
i. Hearing tests		
Glossopharyngeal and Vagus Nerve (CN IX and X)		
i. Palatal and Pharyngeal reflexes (CN IX and X)		
ii. Taste sensation on post 2/3rd of tongue (CN IX)		
iii. History of nasal regurgitation of food		

Spinal-accessory nerve (CN XI)		
i. Flexion of head against resistance		
ii. Rotation of chin		
iii. Shrugging of shoulder		
Hypoglossal nerve (CN XII)		
i. Atrophy of tongue		
ii. Deviation of tongue on protrusion		
iii. Tongue movements		

Result/Interpretation:

Signature of student   *Signature of teacher*

PROFORMA FOR PROCEDURE 10

Subject's name: Date:

Age:

Gender: Male/Female

Does the subject use spectacles: Yes/No

(If yes, mention the refractive index and type of lens)

Tests for vision

		Left eye	*Right eye*
i. Visual acuity			
a. Distant vision	without spectacles		
	with spectacles *(if applicable)*		
b. Near vision	without spectacles		
	with spectacles *(if applicable)*		
ii. Colour vision *(normal/abnormal)*			
iii. Field of vision			
a. Confrontation test *(mention whether normal/restricted in any quadrant)*			
b. Perimetry *(mention the field of vision in degrees in all quadrants).*		Temporal: _____ degrees Inferior: _____ degrees Nasal: _____ degrees Superior: _____ degrees	Temporal: _____ degrees Inferior: _____ degrees Nasal: _____ degrees Superior: _____ degrees

Result/Interpretation:

Signature of student *Signature of teacher*

PROFORMA FOR PROCEDURE 11

Subject's name: Date:

Age:

Gender: Male/Female

Does the subject use hearing aids: Yes/No

If yes, then for which ear: Left ear/Right ear/Both ears

Hearing Tests Assessment

Tests performed	Left ear	Right ear
1. Whisper test (normal/abnormal)		
2. Tuning fork tests		
a. Rinne test (AC>BC or AC<BC)		
b. Weber test (not lateralised or lateralised towards…)		
c. Schwabach test (BC of subject is equal to/ more than/less than examiner)		

Result/Interpretation:

Signature of student   *Signature of teacher*

PROFORMA FOR PROCEDURE 12

Subject's name: Date:

Age:

Gender: Male/Female

Any history of allergy/rhinitis/persistent nasal blockade: Yes/No

Is the subject having common cold: Yes/No

Tests for Olfactory Perception
(*Results to be reported as perceived/not perceived)

Odorant used	Left nostril	Right nostril
1. Peppermint oil		
2. Clove oil		
3. Any other _____ (please specify)		

Result/Interpretation:

Signature of student   *Signature of teacher*

PROFORMA FOR PROCEDURE 13

Subject's name: Date:

Age:

Gender: Male/Female

Tests for Gustatory Perception

Taste sample	Findings (Perceived/Not perceived)
1. Sweet solution	
2. Salt solution	
3. Sour solution	
4. Bitter solution	

Result/Interpretation:

Signature of student   *Signature of teacher*

Notes

Notes

Notes

Notes

Notes

Notes

Certificate of Completion

This is to certify that Mr/Ms _____ roll no _____

has been thoroughly trained in all the 13 clinical procedures contained in the physiology section of the latest Competency

Based Medical Education (CBME) curriculum recommended by Board of Governors, Medical Council of India (MCI).

Henceforth he/she is competent to perform these procedures independently.

His/her overall performance during the year 20_____ –20_____ was average/satisfactory/good/excellent.

_____

Signature of Head
Department of Physiology
(with official seal)

_____

Date